This Medical Journal Belongs To:

MEDICAL CONTACTS

NAME:	**NAME:**	**NAME:**
PHONE:	**PHONE:**	**PHONE:**
EMAIL:	**EMAIL:**	**EMAIL:**
ADDRESS:	**ADDRESS:**	**ADDRESS:**
NAME:	**NAME:**	**NAME:**
PHONE:	**PHONE:**	**PHONE:**
EMAIL:	**EMAIL:**	**EMAIL:**
ADDRESS:	**ADDRESS:**	**ADDRESS:**
NAME:	**NAME:**	**NAME:**
PHONE:	**PHONE:**	**PHONE:**
EMAIL:	**EMAIL:**	**EMAIL:**
ADDRESS:	**ADDRESS:**	**ADDRESS:**

NOTES:

MEDICAL HISTORY

NAME:	BIRTH DATE:
ALLERGIES:	BLOOD TYPE:
FAMILY DOCTOR:	CONTACT:
MEDICATIONS:	

DATE:	IMMUNIZATIONS, SURGERIES, ETC	NOTES:

FAMILY MEDICAL OVERVIEW

HEALTH INSURANCE INFORMATION

DENTAL INSURANCE INFORMATION

OTHER INSURANCE INFORMATION

OTHER INSURANCE INFORMATION

IMPORTANT INFORMATION

ALLERGIES

WHAT: WHO:

BLOOD TYPES

NAME: BLOOD TYPE:

FAMILY DOCTORS

FAMILY DOCTOR
- NAME:
- ADDRESS:
- PHONE:
- ADDITIONAL INFORMATION:

FAMILY DENTIST
- NAME:
- ADDRESS:
- PHONE:
- ADDITIONAL INFORMATION:

OPTOMETRIST
- NAME:
- ADDRESS:
- PHONE:
- ADDITIONAL INFORMATION:

PEDIATRICIAN
- NAME:
- ADDRESS:
- PHONE:
- ADDITIONAL INFORMATION:

VETERINARIAN
- NAME:
- ADDRESS:
- PHONE:
- ADDITIONAL INFORMATION:

MEDICAL CHECKUPS

MONTH:	MONTH:	MONTH:
MONTH:	MONTH:	MONTH:
MONTH:	MONTH:	MONTH:

BLOOD PRESSURE

DATE:	TIME:	BLOOD PRESSURE:	PULSE:

BLOOD SUGAR TRACKER

	BEFORE		MEALS	1 HR	2 HRS	3 HRS
MONDAY		B				
		L				
		D				
		S				
TUESDAY		B				
		L				
		D				
		S				
WEDNESDAY		B				
		L				
		D				
		S				
THURSDAY		B				
		L				
		D				
		S				
FRIDAY		B				
		L				
		D				
		S				

BLOOD SUGAR TRACKER

	BEFORE		MEALS	1 HR	2 HRS	3 HRS
SATURDAY		B				
		L				
		D				
		S				
SUNDAY		B				
		L				
		D				
		S				

NOTES

MEDICATIONS

NAME: **MONTH:**

MEDICATION:	USED FOR:	DOSE:	TIMES P/ DAY:

SURGERIES

NAME: **DATE:**

DATE:	DOCTOR:	REASON:	RESULTS:

IMMUNIZATIONS

NAME:

DATE:	**TYPE:**	**PURPOSE:**	**DOCTOR:**

DOCTOR VISITS

NAME:

DATE:	DOCTOR:	REASON:	RESULTS:

EXAM TRACKER

NAME:	DATE:	DOCTOR:	REASON:	NEXT APPT:

NAME:	DATE:	DOCTOR:	REASON:	NEXT APPT:

NAME:	DATE:	DOCTOR:	REASON:	NEXT APPT:

NAME:	DATE:	DOCTOR:	REASON:	NEXT APPT:

ILLNESS TRACKER

DATE:	DESCRIPTION:	DR. VISIT	TREATMENT
		☐	☐
		☐	☐
		☐	☐
		☐	☐
		☐	☐
		☐	☐
		☐	☐
		☐	☐
		☐	☐
		☐	☐
		☐	☐
		☐	☐
		☐	☐
		☐	☐
		☐	☐
		☐	☐
		☐	☐
		☐	☐
		☐	☐
		☐	☐
		☐	☐
		☐	☐

SYMPTOMS TRACKER

DATE:	DESCRIPTION:	DR. VISIT	TREATMENT
		☐	☐
		☐	☐
		☐	☐
		☐	☐
		☐	☐
		☐	☐
		☐	☐
		☐	☐
		☐	☐
		☐	☐
		☐	☐
		☐	☐
		☐	☐
		☐	☐
		☐	☐
		☐	☐
		☐	☐
		☐	☐
		☐	☐
		☐	☐
		☐	☐
		☐	☐
		☐	☐
		☐	☐

DENTAL VISITS

DENTAL RECORDS FOR:

DENTAL OFFICE:

DATE:	DESCRIPTION:	NEXT APPOINTMENT:

MEDICAL APPOINTMENTS

MEDICAL RECORDS FOR:

DOCTOR OFFICE:

DATE: **DESCRIPTION:**   **NEXT APPOINTMENT:**

DOCTOR VISITS

DATE: FOLLOW UP:

DOCTOR:

HOSPITAL:

REASON/PURPOSE:

NOTES:

DATE: FOLLOW UP:

DOCTOR:

HOSPITAL:

REASON/PURPOSE:

NOTES:

TEST RESULTS

PERIOD OF:

DATE:	TEST:	DOCTOR:	PURPOSE:	RESULTS

MONTHLY HEALTH TRACKER

JANUARY	FEBRUARY	MARCH

APRIL	MAY	JUNE

MONTHLY HEALTH TRACKER

JULY	AUGUST	SEPTEMBER

OCTOBER	NOVEMBER	DECEMBER

YEARLY HEALTH TRACKER

YEAR:

JANUARY	FEBRUARY	MARCH
APRIL	MAY	JUNE
JULY	AUGUST	SEPTEMBER
OCTOBER	NOVEMBER	DECEMBER

NOTES:

MEDICAL EXPENSES

YEAR:

DATE:	DESCRIPTION:	INSURANCE %:	COST:

Notes

MEDICAL CHECKUPS

MONTH:

MONTH:

MONTH:

MONTH:

MONTH:

MONTH:

MONTH:

MONTH:

MONTH:

BLOOD PRESSURE

DATE:	TIME:	BLOOD PRESSURE:	PULSE:

BLOOD SUGAR TRACKER

	BEFORE		MEALS	1 HR	2 HRS	3 HRS
MONDAY		B				
		L				
		D				
		S				
TUESDAY		B				
		L				
		D				
		S				
WEDNESDAY		B				
		L				
		D				
		S				
THURSDAY		B				
		L				
		D				
		S				
FRIDAY		B				
		L				
		D				
		S				

BLOOD SUGAR TRACKER

	BEFORE		MEALS	1 HR	2 HRS	3 HRS
SATURDAY		B				
		L				
		D				
		S				
SUNDAY		B				
		L				
		D				
		S				

NOTES

MEDICATIONS

NAME: **MONTH:**

MEDICATION: **USED FOR:** **DOSE:** **TIMES P/ DAY:**

SURGERIES

NAME: **DATE:**

DATE:	DOCTOR:	REASON:	RESULTS:

IMMUNIZATIONS

NAME:

DATE:	**TYPE:**	**PURPOSE:**	**DOCTOR:**

DOCTOR VISITS

NAME:

DATE:	DOCTOR:	REASON:	RESULTS:

EXAM TRACKER

NAME:	DATE:	DOCTOR:	REASON:	NEXT APPT:

ILLNESS TRACKER

DATE:	DESCRIPTION:	DR. VISIT	TREATMENT
		☐	☐
		☐	☐
		☐	☐
		☐	☐
		☐	☐
		☐	☐
		☐	☐
		☐	☐
		☐	☐
		☐	☐
		☐	☐
		☐	☐
		☐	☐
		☐	☐
		☐	☐
		☐	☐
		☐	☐
		☐	☐
		☐	☐
		☐	☐
		☐	☐
		☐	☐

SYMPTOMS TRACKER

DATE:	DESCRIPTION:	DR. VISIT	TREATMENT
		☐	☐
		☐	☐
		☐	☐
		☐	☐
		☐	☐
		☐	☐
		☐	☐
		☐	☐
		☐	☐
		☐	☐
		☐	☐
		☐	☐
		☐	☐
		☐	☐
		☐	☐
		☐	☐
		☐	☐
		☐	☐
		☐	☐
		☐	☐
		☐	☐
		☐	☐
		☐	☐
		☐	☐

DENTAL VISITS

DENTAL RECORDS FOR:

DENTAL OFFICE:

DATE:	DESCRIPTION:	NEXT APPOINTMENT:

MEDICAL APPOINTMENTS

MEDICAL RECORDS FOR:

DOCTOR OFFICE:

DATE:	DESCRIPTION:	NEXT APPOINTMENT:

DOCTOR VISITS

DATE: FOLLOW UP:

DOCTOR:

HOSPITAL:

REASON/PURPOSE:

NOTES:

DATE: FOLLOW UP:

DOCTOR:

HOSPITAL:

REASON/PURPOSE:

NOTES:

TEST RESULTS

PERIOD OF:

DATE:	TEST:	DOCTOR:	PURPOSE:	RESULTS

MONTHLY HEALTH TRACKER

JANUARY	FEBRUARY	MARCH

APRIL	MAY	JUNE

MONTHLY HEALTH TRACKER

JULY	AUGUST	SEPTEMBER

OCTOBER	NOVEMBER	DECEMBER

YEARLY HEALTH TRACKER

YEAR: _____

JANUARY

FEBRUARY

MARCH

APRIL

MAY

JUNE

JULY

AUGUST

SEPTEMBER

OCTOBER

NOVEMBER

DECEMBER

NOTES:

MEDICAL EXPENSES

YEAR:

DATE:	DESCRIPTION:	INSURANCE %:	COST:

MEDICAL CHECKUPS

☐ MONTH:

☐ MONTH:

☐ MONTH:

☐ MONTH:

☐ MONTH:

☐ MONTH:

☐ MONTH:

☐ MONTH:

☐ MONTH:

BLOOD PRESSURE

DATE: **TIME:** **BLOOD PRESSURE:** **PULSE:**

BLOOD SUGAR TRACKER

	BEFORE		MEALS	1 HR	2 HRS	3 HRS
MONDAY		B				
		L				
		D				
		S				
TUESDAY		B				
		L				
		D				
		S				
WEDNESDAY		B				
		L				
		D				
		S				
THURSDAY		B				
		L				
		D				
		S				
FRIDAY		B				
		L				
		D				
		S				

BLOOD SUGAR TRACKER

BEFORE		MEALS	1 HR	2 HRS	3 HRS
SATURDAY	B L D S				
SUNDAY	B L D S				

NOTES

MEDICATIONS

NAME: **MONTH:**

MEDICATION:	USED FOR:	DOSE:	TIMES P/ DAY:

SURGERIES

NAME: **DATE:**

DATE: **DOCTOR:** **REASON:** **RESULTS:**

IMMUNIZATIONS

NAME:

DATE:	TYPE:	PURPOSE:	DOCTOR:

DOCTOR VISITS

NAME:

DATE:	DOCTOR:	REASON:	RESULTS:

EXAM TRACKER

NAME:	DATE:	DOCTOR:	REASON:	NEXT APPT:

NAME:	DATE:	DOCTOR:	REASON:	NEXT APPT:

NAME:	DATE:	DOCTOR:	REASON:	NEXT APPT:

NAME:	DATE:	DOCTOR:	REASON:	NEXT APPT:

ILLNESS TRACKER

DATE: **DESCRIPTION:** DR. VISIT TREATMENT

SYMPTOMS TRACKER

DATE:	DESCRIPTION:	DR. VISIT	TREATMENT
		☐	☐
		☐	☐
		☐	☐
		☐	☐
		☐	☐
		☐	☐
		☐	☐
		☐	☐
		☐	☐
		☐	☐
		☐	☐
		☐	☐
		☐	☐
		☐	☐
		☐	☐
		☐	☐
		☐	☐
		☐	☐
		☐	☐
		☐	☐
		☐	☐
		☐	☐
		☐	☐

DENTAL VISITS

DENTAL RECORDS FOR:

DENTAL OFFICE:

| DATE: | DESCRIPTION: | NEXT APPOINTMENT: |

MEDICAL APPOINTMENTS

MEDICAL RECORDS FOR:

DOCTOR OFFICE:

DATE:	DESCRIPTION:	NEXT APPOINTMENT:

DOCTOR VISITS

DATE: FOLLOW UP:

DOCTOR:

HOSPITAL:

REASON/PURPOSE:

NOTES:

DATE: FOLLOW UP:

DOCTOR:

HOSPITAL:

REASON/PURPOSE:

NOTES:

TEST RESULTS

PERIOD OF:

DATE:	TEST:	DOCTOR:	PURPOSE:	RESULTS

MONTHLY HEALTH TRACKER

JANUARY	FEBRUARY	MARCH

APRIL	MAY	JUNE

MONTHLY HEALTH TRACKER

JULY	AUGUST	SEPTEMBER

OCTOBER	NOVEMBER	DECEMBER

YEARLY HEALTH TRACKER

YEAR: _____

JANUARY

FEBRUARY

MARCH

APRIL

MAY

JUNE

JULY

AUGUST

SEPTEMBER

OCTOBER

NOVEMBER

DECEMBER

NOTES:

MEDICAL EXPENSES

YEAR:

DATE:	DESCRIPTION:	INSURANCE %:	COST:

Notes

MEDICAL CHECKUPS

☐ MONTH:	☐ MONTH:	☐ MONTH:
☐ MONTH:	☐ MONTH:	☐ MONTH:
☐ MONTH:	☐ MONTH:	☐ MONTH:

BLOOD PRESSURE

DATE: **TIME:** **BLOOD PRESSURE:** **PULSE:**

BLOOD SUGAR TRACKER

	BEFORE		MEALS	1 HR	2 HRS	3 HRS
MONDAY		B				
		L				
		D				
		S				
TUESDAY		B				
		L				
		D				
		S				
WEDNESDAY		B				
		L				
		D				
		S				
THURSDAY		B				
		L				
		D				
		S				
FRIDAY		B				
		L				
		D				
		S				

BLOOD SUGAR TRACKER

BEFORE		MEALS	1 HR	2 HRS	3 HRS
SATURDAY	B L D S				
SUNDAY	B L D S				

NOTES

MEDICATIONS

NAME: **MONTH:**

MEDICATION:	USED FOR:	DOSE:	TIMES P/ DAY:

SURGERIES

NAME: **DATE:**

DATE:	DOCTOR:	REASON:	RESULTS:

IMMUNIZATIONS

NAME:

DATE:	TYPE:	PURPOSE:	DOCTOR:

DOCTOR VISITS

NAME:

DATE:	**DOCTOR:**	**REASON:**	**RESULTS:**

EXAM TRACKER

NAME:	DATE:	DOCTOR:	REASON:	NEXT APPT:

NAME:	DATE:	DOCTOR:	REASON:	NEXT APPT:

NAME:	DATE:	DOCTOR:	REASON:	NEXT APPT:

NAME:	DATE:	DOCTOR:	REASON:	NEXT APPT:

ILLNESS TRACKER

DATE: **DESCRIPTION:** **DR. VISIT** **TREATMENT**

SYMPTOMS TRACKER

DATE:	DESCRIPTION:	DR. VISIT	TREATMENT
		☐	☐
		☐	☐
		☐	☐
		☐	☐
		☐	☐
		☐	☐
		☐	☐
		☐	☐
		☐	☐
		☐	☐
		☐	☐
		☐	☐
		☐	☐
		☐	☐
		☐	☐
		☐	☐
		☐	☐
		☐	☐
		☐	☐
		☐	☐
		☐	☐
		☐	☐

DENTAL VISITS

DENTAL RECORDS FOR:

DENTAL OFFICE:

DATE: DESCRIPTION: NEXT APPOINTMENT:

MEDICAL APPOINTMENTS

MEDICAL RECORDS FOR:

DOCTOR OFFICE:

DATE:	DESCRIPTION:	NEXT APPOINTMENT:

DOCTOR VISITS

DATE:					FOLLOW UP:

DOCTOR:

HOSPITAL:

REASON/PURPOSE:

NOTES:

DATE:					FOLLOW UP:

DOCTOR:

HOSPITAL:

REASON/PURPOSE:

NOTES:

TEST RESULTS

PERIOD OF:

DATE:	TEST:	DOCTOR:	PURPOSE:	RESULTS

MONTHLY HEALTH TRACKER

JANUARY	FEBRUARY	MARCH

APRIL	MAY	JUNE

MONTHLY HEALTH TRACKER

JULY	AUGUST	SEPTEMBER

OCTOBER	NOVEMBER	DECEMBER

YEARLY HEALTH TRACKER

YEAR: _____

JANUARY   **FEBRUARY**   **MARCH**

APRIL   **MAY**   **JUNE**

JULY   **AUGUST**   **SEPTEMBER**

OCTOBER   **NOVEMBER**   **DECEMBER**

NOTES:

MEDICAL EXPENSES

YEAR:

DATE:	DESCRIPTION:	INSURANCE %:	COST:

Notes

MEDICAL CHECKUPS

☐ MONTH:	☐ MONTH:	☐ MONTH:
☐ MONTH:	☐ MONTH:	☐ MONTH:
☐ MONTH:	☐ MONTH:	☐ MONTH:

BLOOD PRESSURE

DATE: **TIME:** **BLOOD PRESSURE:** **PULSE:**

BLOOD SUGAR TRACKER

	BEFORE		MEALS	1 HR	2 HRS	3 HRS
MONDAY		B				
		L				
		D				
		S				
TUESDAY		B				
		L				
		D				
		S				
WEDNESDAY		B				
		L				
		D				
		S				
THURSDAY		B				
		L				
		D				
		S				
FRIDAY		B				
		L				
		D				
		S				

BLOOD SUGAR TRACKER

	BEFORE	MEALS		1 HR	2 HRS	3 HRS
SATURDAY		B				
		L				
		D				
		S				
SUNDAY		B				
		L				
		D				
		S				

NOTES

MEDICATIONS

NAME: **MONTH:**

MEDICATION:	USED FOR:	DOSE:	TIMES P/ DAY:

SURGERIES

NAME: **DATE:**

DATE: **DOCTOR:** **REASON:** **RESULTS:**

IMMUNIZATIONS

NAME:

DATE:	TYPE:	PURPOSE:	DOCTOR:

DOCTOR VISITS

NAME:

DATE:	**DOCTOR:**	**REASON:**	**RESULTS:**

EXAM TRACKER

NAME:	DATE:	DOCTOR:	REASON:	NEXT APPT:

NAME:	DATE:	DOCTOR:	REASON:	NEXT APPT:

NAME:	DATE:	DOCTOR:	REASON:	NEXT APPT:

NAME:	DATE:	DOCTOR:	REASON:	NEXT APPT:

ILLNESS TRACKER

DATE: **DESCRIPTION:** DR. VISIT TREATMENT

SYMPTOMS TRACKER

DATE:	DESCRIPTION:	DR. VISIT	TREATMENT
		☐	☐
		☐	☐
		☐	☐
		☐	☐
		☐	☐
		☐	☐
		☐	☐
		☐	☐
		☐	☐
		☐	☐
		☐	☐
		☐	☐
		☐	☐
		☐	☐
		☐	☐
		☐	☐
		☐	☐
		☐	☐
		☐	☐
		☐	☐
		☐	☐

DENTAL VISITS

DENTAL RECORDS FOR:

DENTAL OFFICE:

| DATE: | DESCRIPTION: | NEXT APPOINTMENT: |

MEDICAL APPOINTMENTS

MEDICAL RECORDS FOR:

DOCTOR OFFICE:

DATE:	DESCRIPTION:	NEXT APPOINTMENT:

DOCTOR VISITS

DATE:

DOCTOR:

HOSPITAL:

REASON/PURPOSE:

NOTES:

FOLLOW UP:

DATE:

DOCTOR:

HOSPITAL:

REASON/PURPOSE:

NOTES:

FOLLOW UP:

TEST RESULTS

PERIOD OF:

DATE:	TEST:	DOCTOR:	PURPOSE:	RESULTS

MONTHLY HEALTH TRACKER

JANUARY	FEBRUARY	MARCH

APRIL	MAY	JUNE

MONTHLY HEALTH TRACKER

JULY	AUGUST	SEPTEMBER

OCTOBER	NOVEMBER	DECEMBER

YEARLY HEALTH TRACKER

YEAR: _____

JANUARY   FEBRUARY   MARCH

APRIL   MAY   JUNE

JULY   AUGUST   SEPTEMBER

OCTOBER   NOVEMBER   DECEMBER

NOTES:

MEDICAL EXPENSES

YEAR:

DATE:	DESCRIPTION:	INSURANCE %:	COST:

MEDICAL CHECKUPS

MONTH:	MONTH:	MONTH:
MONTH:	MONTH:	MONTH:
MONTH:	MONTH:	MONTH:

BLOOD PRESSURE

DATE:	TIME:	BLOOD PRESSURE:	PULSE:

BLOOD SUGAR TRACKER

	BEFORE		MEALS	1 HR	2 HRS	3 HRS
MONDAY		B				
		L				
		D				
		S				
TUESDAY		B				
		L				
		D				
		S				
WEDNESDAY		B				
		L				
		D				
		S				
THURSDAY		B				
		L				
		D				
		S				
FRIDAY		B				
		L				
		D				
		S				

BLOOD SUGAR TRACKER

BEFORE		MEALS	1 HR	2 HRS	3 HRS
SATURDAY	B				
	L				
	D				
	S				
SUNDAY	B				
	L				
	D				
	S				

NOTES

MEDICATIONS

NAME: **MONTH:**

MEDICATION: **USED FOR:** **DOSE:** **TIMES P/ DAY:**

IMMUNIZATIONS

NAME:

DATE:	TYPE:	PURPOSE:	DOCTOR:

DOCTOR VISITS

NAME:

DATE:	**DOCTOR:**	**REASON:**	**RESULTS:**

SYMPTOMS TRACKER

DATE:	DESCRIPTION:	DR. VISIT	TREATMENT
		☐	☐
		☐	☐
		☐	☐
		☐	☐
		☐	☐
		☐	☐
		☐	☐
		☐	☐
		☐	☐
		☐	☐
		☐	☐
		☐	☐
		☐	☐
		☐	☐
		☐	☐
		☐	☐
		☐	☐
		☐	☐
		☐	☐
		☐	☐
		☐	☐
		☐	☐

MEDICAL APPOINTMENTS

MEDICAL RECORDS FOR:

DOCTOR OFFICE:

DATE:	DESCRIPTION:	NEXT APPOINTMENT:

DOCTOR VISITS

DATE:

FOLLOW UP:

DOCTOR:

HOSPITAL:

REASON/PURPOSE:

NOTES:

DATE:

FOLLOW UP:

DOCTOR:

HOSPITAL:

REASON/PURPOSE:

NOTES:

TEST RESULTS

PERIOD OF:

DATE: **TEST:** **DOCTOR:** **PURPOSE:** **RESULTS**

MONTHLY HEALTH TRACKER

JANUARY	FEBRUARY	MARCH

APRIL	MAY	JUNE

MONTHLY HEALTH TRACKER

JULY	AUGUST	SEPTEMBER

OCTOBER	NOVEMBER	DECEMBER

BLOOD PRESSURE

DATE:	TIME:	BLOOD PRESSURE:	PULSE:

BLOOD SUGAR TRACKER

BEFORE		MEALS	1 HR	2 HRS	3 HRS
MONDAY	B				
	L				
	D				
	S				
TUESDAY	B				
	L				
	D				
	S				
WEDNESDAY	B				
	L				
	D				
	S				
THURSDAY	B				
	L				
	D				
	S				
FRIDAY	B				
	L				
	D				
	S				

BLOOD SUGAR TRACKER

	BEFORE		MEALS	1 HR	2 HRS	3 HRS
SATURDAY		B				
		L				
		D				
		S				
SUNDAY		B				
		L				
		D				
		S				

NOTES

www.ingramcontent.com/pod-product-compliance
Lightning Source LLC
Chambersburg PA
CBHW080549220526
45466CB00010B/3093